Zoltan Rona MD MSc

Menopause
Normally and Naturally

The truth about hormone replacement therapy and more

books

Vancouver
Canada

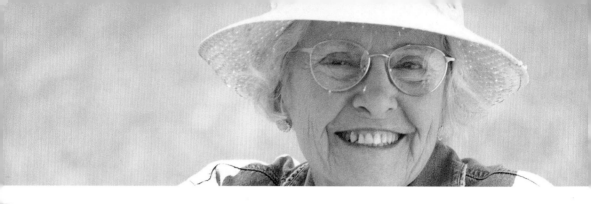

Contents

Note: Conversions in this book (from imperial to metric) are not exact. They have been rounded to the nearest measurement for convenience. Exact measurements are given in imperial. The recipes in this book are by no means to be taken as therapeutic. They simply promote the philosophy of both the author and alive books in relation to whole foods, health and nutrition, while incorporating the practical advice given by the author in the first section of the book.

Recipes

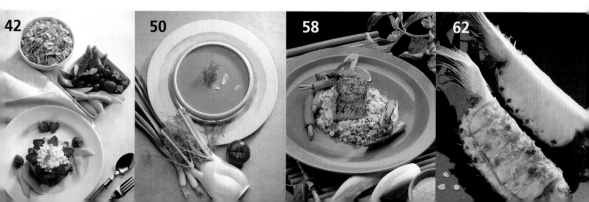

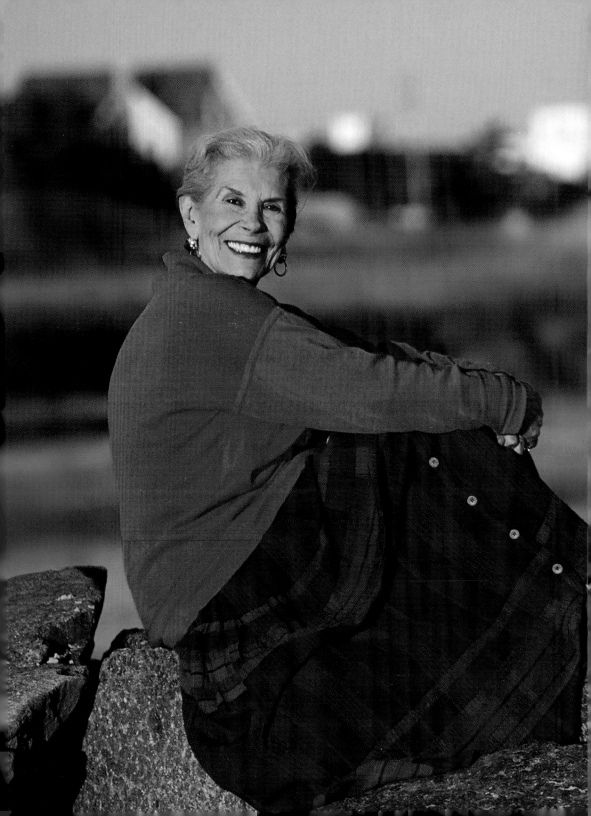

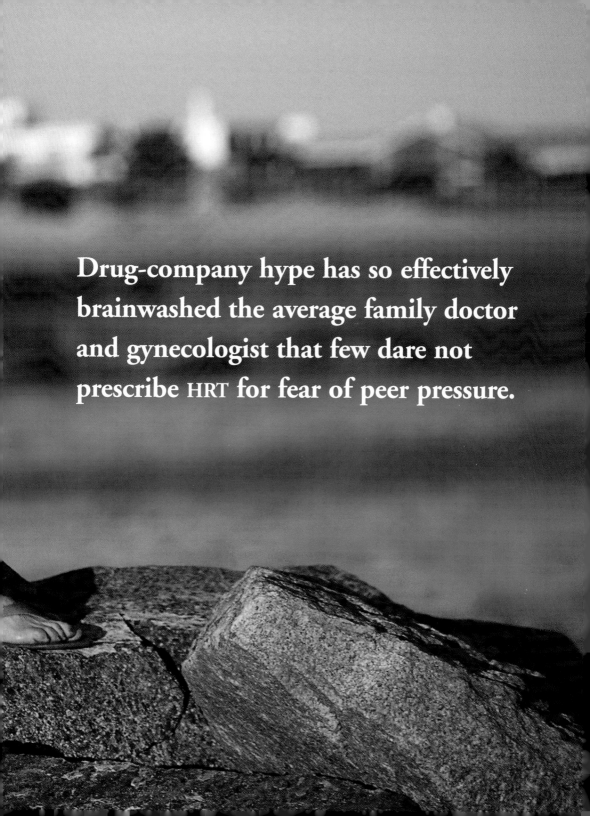

Drug-company hype has so effectively brainwashed the average family doctor and gynecologist that few dare not prescribe HRT for fear of peer pressure.

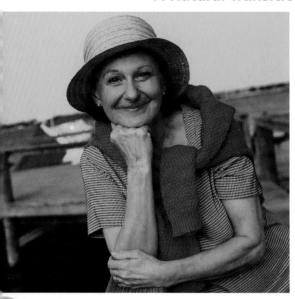

Women who reject the medicalization of menopause are opting for a natural approach.

One of the major reasons why women in their late forties or early fifties seek out a natural health care practitioner like myself is to get advice about what they should or should not be doing about menopause. Many women are confused and worried by what they see and hear in the media. And they are not helped by the conventional medical community, which, for the most part, still sees menopause as a hormone deficiency syndrome requiring diagnosis and treatment. They argue that menopausal women are at increased risk for developing heart disease, bone loss (osteoporosis), breast cancer and endometrial cancer. They believe that the risk of developing some of these diseases can be reduced by treating women with hormone replacement therapy (HRT) made up of synthetic estrogen and progesterone. In fact, from what many of my patients tell me, doctors employ high-pressure psychological tactics including outright lies in order to convince women to use HRT. Drug company hype has so effectively brainwashed the average family doctor and gynecologist that few dare not prescribe HRT for fear of peer pressure.

> **Does this sound familiar?**
> Dr. A: "If you do not take estrogen, you will be a heart attack waiting to happen."
> Dr. B: "Without HRT you will dry up like a prune and get osteoporosis just like your mother did."
> Dr. C: "There is no proof that any of those herbs or vitamins help hot flashes. The only thing they do is create expensive urine. They might even be toxic to your liver. Only HRT has been proven to get rid of hot flashes safely and prevent both heart disease and cancer."

Women have been subjected to this HRT dogma for at least the past two decades. A growing number, however, are opting for a different approach to menopause through the use of natural hormone replacement therapy (NHRT), which involves the use of dietary modification and the supplementation of various vitamins, minerals, and herbal remedies.

Many women are opting for this natural approach because they reject the medicalization of menopause. After all, isn't the change of life a normal event in all women's lives? Rather than a loss of youth that needs to be reversed by HRT, why not welcome menopause as the beginning of a new freedom from menstrual cycles and reproductive responsibilities? Life after menopause can be a very positive experience, according to anthropologist Margaret Mead, who used the term "postmenopausal zest" to describe the surge of physical and psychological energy that many women feel at this time.

Women entering menopause should be looking forward to a vigorous, worry-free, active, and healthy middle and old age. Many women will live thirty years (one-third of their lives) after menopause: to ensure that these "golden" years are enjoyed to the fullest, women must make conscious efforts to improve and build their health in the years leading up to menopause. And there is a lot a woman can do nutritionally to prepare for menopause and in the process build upon the health that will sustain her for the rest of her life.

Most importantly, women must take more responsibility for their health through self-education, through consultation with a health care provider who is sympathetic to their concerns, and by questioning the mainstream dogma that would have women take drugs for what is a natural life transition. This said, I do not discount those women for whom menopause presents some very real concerns. This book will offer women who are committed to HRT some natural ways of preventing some of the

Many women turn to natural healthcare options for menopause because they do not get the help or answers they require from the conventional medical community.

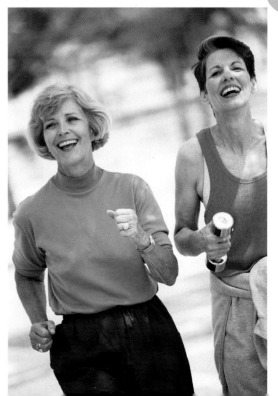

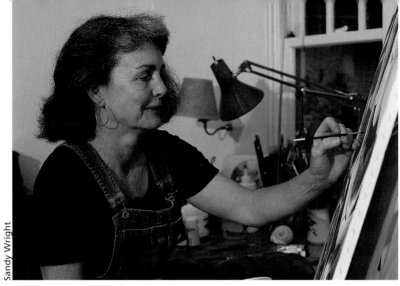

Sandy Wright

All women can and will get through the challenges posed by menopause without having to do anything drastic about it.

side effects or long-term complications of synthetic estrogen and progesterone.

The message I am hoping to convey with this book is that virtually all women can and will get through the challenges posed by menopause without having to do anything drastic about it. There is no dire urgency to see doctors, use HRT, water pills, tranquilizers, or worry about suddenly succumbing to a long list of diseases for which only drugs and surgery are the cure.

This is not to say that women should blindly go about their lives as if nothing is happening; rather, I want to emphasis that menopause is not an abnormal condition that requires medication and numerous doctor visits. Menopause is one of life's transitions, as is birth and death.

The media and medical industry has had the effect of making women think that menopause is a negative thing that should somehow be suppressed, drugged, or stopped. My advice is to ignore this sales job and focus on the many positive aspects of menopause. Just think of it—no more periods, no more fears of getting pregnant. No need for strange and unpleasant forms of birth control. For some women plagued with uterine fibroids, migraine headaches and painful periods, menopause brings an end to years of suffering.

Moreover, menopause can be a significant health-enhancing event in a woman's life. It presents an opportunity for a woman to reacquaint herself with her body and take control of her health by making diet and lifestyle changes. A better diet and a few natural vitamin and mineral supplements may be all that's necessary for most women to feel at their best. Others might need to use one or more of the herbal remedies discussed in this book in addition to that. Very few will actually need to take hormones, natural or otherwise, for any length of time to get through the transition.

If you do need to see a doctor for menopausal concerns, visit one who sees the change as a natural life event and not as a disease requiring HRT as a cure. Naturopaths and holistic medical doctors are the best types of doctors to visit in this regard but a growing number of conventional doctors are adopting this more enlightened attitude as well. In Toronto, where I practice, I know of at least two gynecologists who rarely prescribe HRT and tend to rely on common sense, advising women about a healthy diet and a few nutritional supplements. This will be the way in which all health care professionals view menopause in the future. You need not wait for this to happen before acting on your own to practice the preventive and natural approaches discussed in this book.

What is Menopause? . . . .

Menopause, or "the change of life," is the time in a woman's life when menstruation stops permanently. The ovaries reduce their production of female sex hormones, a gradual process that begins about three to five years (or longer for some women) before the final menstrual period. These transitional years are referred to as the "climacteric" or "perimenopause."

Menopause is considered complete or finished (post-menopause) when a woman has been without periods for one year. The average age at which this occurs is fifty but this number is variable from woman to woman. Menopause starts around the late forties when periods start to get more irregular, and finally stop altogether at an average age of fifty (earlier in black and non-European women).

Menopause is when a woman's ovaries reduce their production of female sex hormones, and menstruation stops permanently.

9

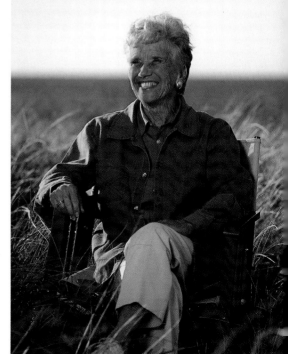

Artificial menopause is that which is brought about by the surgical excision of a woman's ovaries due to medical reasons (endometriosis, fibroids, cancer of the uterus, for example). Women who have undergone the surgical removal of their ovaries (a hysterectomy) usually experience a more uncomfortable form of menopause, and are at a greater risk for heart disease as well as osteoporosis and depression.

Menopause, if not precipitated by such surgery, is a natural event in every woman's life. It is not a "deficiency disease" or "deterioration," or any other of the long list of archaic, patriarchal medical labels. It is a process of change and transition as a woman's body sheds its childbearing potential and adjusts to lower levels of hormones.

In the healthy female, once the ovaries stop producing the female hormones, the adrenal glands eventually produce enough hormones to maintain balance. During this transition period, women experience a host of symptoms that prompt them to visit their doctors. Unfortunately, such doctor visits in North America all too often end with a prescription for hormones that have a long list of hazardous side effects.

Risk Factor Associated with Hormone Replacement Therapy

Among many side effects (see page 21), the use of estrogen hormone by itself is associated with a three- to four-times greater incidence of uterine cancer. To lower the potential cancer risk, doctors usually add a progesterone prescription for ten days out of every cycle. Unfortunately, this causes menopausal women to continue to bleed monthly after menopause; this will continue as long as hormone replacement therapy is used.

Hormone replacement therapy is also linked to an increased risk of breast cancer. According to Dr. Sidney Wolfe and a 1991 article in the *Journal of the American Medical Association,* "If a woman used estrogen pills for fifteen years, she had a 30 percent excess rate of breast cancer. If used for twenty-five years, a "goal" toward which many doctors are pushing their patients, there would be a 50 percent increased risk of breast cancer." Women have now been exposed to both long-term hormone treatment in the form of the birth control pill, and long-term hormone treatment in the form of estrogen replacement for close to three decades. And no one really knows what the combined effect might be on the intricate workings of the female reproductive system.

Menopausal symptoms can be controlled naturally and without any significant side effects. Moreover, osteoporosis and coronary artery disease can be prevented and even reversed by diet and lifestyle changes alone.

Menopause is an individualized experience with nothing about it cast in stone. Some women welcome the prospect of having no more menstrual periods, notice little to no difference in their bodies or moods and cannot understand what all the fuss is about. Others find the change of life so extremely bothersome and disruptive that they feel their life will suddenly come to an abrupt end. And indeed, the effects of a lower level of estrogen and progesterone, while not identical from woman to woman, can produce several discomforts, at various levels of severity.

The Adrenal Gland Connection . . . .

Menopause is one major life event strongly connected to adrenal glandular function. In the healthy female, once the ovaries stop producing estrogen and progesterone, the adrenal glands take over production to maintain a comfortable balance. If this transition period does not occur smoothly, women entering menopause will experience severe and often debilitating hot flashes, vaginal dryness, depression, loss of libido, accelerating osteoporosis, memory disturbances and blood sugar control problems (hypoglycemia). Adrenal insufficiency can cause exaggerated or early

Stress–both emotional and physical–weakens the adrenal glands.

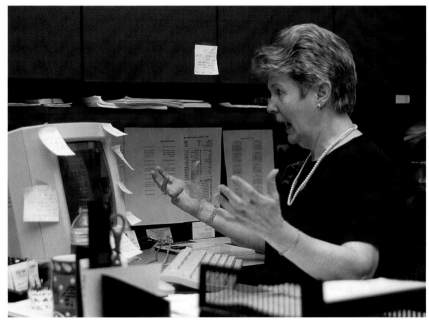

menopausal discomforts that create the illusion that prescription hormone replacement therapy is needed. Indeed, the ease with which such transitions take place is highly dependent on the strength of a woman's adrenals and her general state of health. Unfortunately, many women approach menopause with nutritional depletions that have led to less than optimal adrenal function.

How do the Adrenals Weaken?

Most commonly, different types of stress–both physical and emotional–are involved. While some of these stresses are beyond our immediate control, many are dependent on our diet and lifestyle choices. For example, a diet high in refined carbohydrates, as well as heavy consumption of cigarettes, alcohol, and drugs will stress the adrenals by causing a greater than normal secretion of adrenal hormones, leading to eventual depletion of stress hormone reserves. Working long hours under fluorescent lights at a sedentary job and getting little to no exercise also weakens adrenal function.

Conventional medicine categorizes adrenal function as normal, low (adrenal insufficiency, a.k.a. Addison's disease) or high (Cushing's Syndrome, a rare disorder caused by an overactive adrenal cortex). Those affected by suboptimal adrenal function fall between the two extremes and are left without any medical solution to their health problems. If the initial screening tests fail to show either low or high levels of various steroids, reductionistic medical thinking, regardless of patient signs and symptoms, is that adrenal function is normal. However, studies show that adrenal function can be compromised long before abnormalities start appearing in such laboratory tests, and that the use of adrenal glandular support reverses signs and symptoms and replenishes depleted organ reserves.

Signs and Symptoms of Weak Adrenal Function

The many signs and symptoms of adrenal insufficiency are often brushed off by conventional doctors as a case of "nerves" requiring a prescription for antidepressants, tranquilizers or estrogen. Many of these signs and symptoms, however, should alert both doctor and patient to look deeper into organic sources with the use of special tests (e.g., glucose tolerance test, hormone challenge tests). The results of these tests could provide a more definitive diagnosis.

An inability to concentrate, excessive fatigue, nervousness, irritability, depression, and anxiety are the most common symptoms of weak adrenal function.

Progesterone is one of the most important hormones secreted by the adrenal gland. Progesterone has a major role to play in healthy menstruation, bone building, fertility, and menopause. Many women who suffer from hot flashes, vaginal dryness, mood swings and other problems associated with menopause are often suffering from relatively low progesterone levels, which can often be corrected by normalizing adrenal function.

Adrenal Glandular Support

The adrenal gland manufactures the same sex hormones that are made in the ovaries. In healthy premenopausal women there is a balance between the ovaries and the adrenal glands. When ovarian function begins to change in the perimenopausal period the adrenal glands start to make more sex hormones to pick up the slack. If the adrenal glands are stressed they may not be capable of making enough of the sex hormones to compensate for

Incorporating deep-water ocean fish, such as salmon, in the diet will support adrenal function.

13

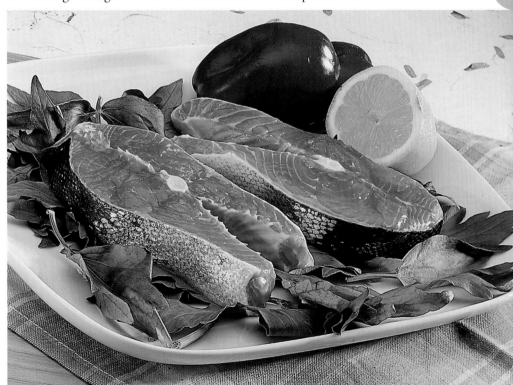

weakened or completely inactive ovaries. Thus, the health of the adrenal glands may be crucial for women who want to prevent or lessen some of the discomfort that occurs both before and during menopause. Happily, adrenal function can be improved with a combination of diet and lifestyle changes.

Diet: Avoid foods and beverages that unnecessarily stress the adrenals, especially alcohol, caffeine, tobacco, fried foods, processed foods, sugar, and refined carbohydrates. A high percentage of symptomatic individuals are allergic to gluten (wheat, spelt, rye, barley, oats) and casein (dairy products) and should avoid these foods altogether. Unless allergic to them, eat more deep-water ocean fish, salmon, tuna, trout, fresh fruits, and green leafy vegetables, garlic, onions, shiitake or maitake mushrooms, and legumes.

Lifestyle: Emotional or psychological stress stimulates the adrenal glands to make more adrenalin, cortisol, and sex hormones, all of which can give both the mind and body some protection and ammunition to deal effectively with whatever the stress presents to the individual. If emotional or psychological stress persists or becomes chronic, the ability of the adrenal glands to manufacture these hormones eventually becomes unable to keep pace with the seemingly endless stress. People experiencing this phenomenon describe themselves as suffering from "burnout." If the fuel to combat stress is no longer available it's very much like driving a car without oil or gasoline. The emotional or psychological stress is still there but the ability to compensate for it is no longer is possible. Depression, chronic fatigue, chronic pain, and a long list of physical and psychological symptoms develop.

The best way of allowing the adrenal glands to recover is to remove the stressor or stressors. This may not always be possible, but the damaging effects of stress can be at least blunted. There are many ways of refueling the adrenal glands using stress-reducing techniques. Some women will find that rest, time off work, or daily aerobic exercise help. Others will benefit from meditation, prayer, psychotherapy, biofeedback, yoga, massage therapy, or some combination thereof. A healthier diet, nutritional supplements and herbal supplements will also help with stress reduction.

Nutritional and Herbal Supplements

The following supplements will provide support for weakened adrenals. (Dosages are dependent on severity of symptoms and individual tolerances. Consult your health care practitioner.)

Multiple vitamin and mineral supplement

Green drink (spirulina, chlorella, barley, kamut, etc.)

Bee pollen or royal jelly

B-complex vitamins with extra vitamin B_5 (pantothenic acid)

Vitamin C and bioflavonoids

Raw adrenal extract

Raw liver extract

Coenzyme Q_{10}

Astragalus

Echinacea

Licorice root

Milk thistle

Siberian ginseng

Physical Discomforts of Menopause . . . .

There are at least thirty-five different symptoms (discomforts) generally associated with menopause, most of which can be divided into two subcategories: physical and mental. Most women, however, only suffer from one or two major discomforts, and it is these that compel them to seek professional advice. The discomforts are all due to the gradually diminishing levels of estrogen, progesterone, DHEA and testosterone by the ovaries without adequate compensation by the adrenal glands to make up for the low hormone levels.

Symptoms are highly variable in terms of number and severity from one woman to the next. For some, the problems are so severe that they may not be able to go to work. For others, menopause will be a barely

Among the most distressing of problems associated with menopause is "hot flashes" or "night sweats."

15

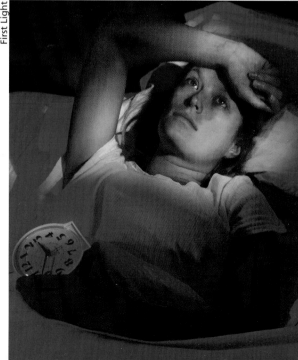
First Light

noticeable event other than for the loss of monthly periods. The following is a list of problems that have been reported by women during menopause, starting with the most common:

Hot flashes, flushes, night sweats and/or cold flashes; clammy feeling

These may be the most distressing of all the problems encountered by women during menopause. They are also the symptoms for which doctors most often prescribe hormones and tranquilizers.

Bouts of rapid heartbeat

These symptoms are related to hot flashes but may occur without hot flashes. Though annoying, they are not usually a sign of a significant health problem.

Irregular periods; shorter, lighter, or heavier periods; shorter or longer cycles

The occurrence of these scenarios depends largely on the relative levels of estrogen and progesterone.

Dry vagina and painful intercourse

This is directly attributable to low estrogen levels. Although many women can benefit from natural therapies with various herbs, many require prescription estrogen creams to get adequate relief.

Overwhelming fatigue

If this is a problem, look at adrenal hormone levels (DHEA and cortisol). If adrenal function is weak, some of the natural approaches to adrenal insufficiency can be used (see page 13).

Incontinence, especially upon sneezing or laughing; urge incontinence

These symptoms are an indication of weakened muscle tone, which can sometimes be helped by exercises as well as by HRT and NHRT.

Aching, sore joints, muscles and tendons (may include such problems as carpal tunnel syndrome)

Joint, muscle and tendon problems occur more often because of lower levels of cortisol, DHEA or testosterone, all of which have anti-inflammatory, antiallergy, and antiaging qualities, and muscle strengthening properties.

Breast tenderness

Sore, painful, and lumpy breasts are usually the result of a relatively lower level of progesterone.

Headache change: increase or decrease

Too much estrogen relative to progesterone tends to increase fluid retention, which, if it happens in the brain, increases headaches. When progesterone levels are relatively higher than estrogen levels, headaches tend to decrease because excess fluid retention is prevented.

Worsening medical conditions (high blood pressure, heart disease, diabetes, arthritis)

Low levels of DHEA and testosterone have been linked to most degenerative diseases. While many people accept these health problems as inevitable consequences of aging, normalizing adrenal function will boost levels of these hormones and improve or even reverse the medical conditions.

Increased allergies

This is a symptom generally caused by a low progesterone level because progesterone is needed by the body to manufacture cortisol, an anti-inflammatory and antiallergy hormone.

Weight gain, often around the waist and thighs, resulting in a "disappearing waistline"

Low progesterone, DHEA and testosterone levels allow estrogen from food or environmental chemicals to increase fat deposition in the waist and thighs. In addition, these hormones modulate thyroid hormone activity, which is weakened when progesterone and DHEA levels go too low. Low thyroid activity encourages weight gain.

Hair loss or thinning (head, pubic, or whole body); increase in facial hair

Male pattern baldness in women as well as an increase in facial hair is thought to be due to dihydro-testosterone (DHT), a metabolite of testosterone that increases when progesterone levels are too low. Progesterone keeps DHT under control and prevents these undesirable traits in women.

Thinning skin

Low estrogen, progesterone, testosterone, and DHEA can cause changes to the skin including wrinkling, thinning, and excessive dryness.

Osteoporosis (after several years)

At one time it was thought that only a lack of estrogen and calcium led to osteoporosis. We now know that a lack of other adrenal and ovarian hormones like DHEA and testosterone are also involved.

Menopause and Osteoporosis

Osteoporosis is a potentially serious skeletal disease that affects millions of women after the onset of menopause. It is characterized by a decrease in bone mass due to an imbalance between bone reabsorption and bone formation leading to an increased susceptibility to fractures.

Low estrogen is but one of forty factors involved in the development of osteoporosis. Exercise and a vegetarian (or low protein) diet have been shown to be far more important for osteoporosis prevention than estrogen levels. Other major risk factors for the development of osteoporosis are cigarette smoking, excessive alcohol and caffeine intake, having had the ovaries removed (or other causes of early menopause), a family history of osteoporosis, never having been pregnant, drugs such as cortisone, diuretics (water pills), anti-seizure medications and anticoagulants ("blood thinners"), digestive disorders and overactive endocrine glands (especially hyperthyroidism). A family history of osteoporosis is probably the most reliable indication that an individual is at risk for the condition.

While there are clear-cut advantages to the use of HRT with regards to the prevention of osteoporosis and other effects of aging, the cure may be worse than the disease. For example, HRT has been linked to increasing incidences of breast cancer, high blood pressure, strokes, cardiovascular disease, chronic candida (yeast) infections, abnormal blood clotting problems (thrombosis), migraine headaches, and other undesirable conditions.

Changes in fingernails: softer, crack or break easier

DHEA and testosterone have nourishing (anabolic) effects on not only the muscles and bones but also the nails.

Mental Discomforts of Menopause . . . .

The lower production of hormones that occurs with menopause can cause changes in the brain and nervous system due to the effects of abnormally fluctuating blood sugar levels and a lower activity of thyroid hormone. Progesterone, testosterone, and DHEA stabilize blood sugar levels. A sudden lack of these hormones allows blood sugar levels to soar and then plummet rapidly. Since these hormones also affect the activity of thyroid hormone, a long list of physical, psychological, and emotional changes start showing up. The emotional roller coaster attributed to menopause expresses itself in one or more of the following common complaints:

Irritability
Too much estrogen relative to progesterone tends to increase fluid retention, which, if it happens in the brain, can cause irritability. Low blood sugar levels are another cause of irritability.

Mood swings, depression, sudden tears or temper tantrums
These are common symptoms of either low blood sugar (hypoglycemia) or a low thyroid, both of which occur due to lower levels of adrenal/ovarian hormones.

Trouble sleeping through the night (with or without night sweats)
This, too, is a common symptom of either low blood sugar (hypoglycemia) or a low thyroid.

Loss of libido
This is usually related to low DHEA, testosterone, and/or progesterone levels.

Anxiety, feeling ill at ease
These, too, are common symptoms of either low blood sugar (hypoglycemia) or a low thyroid.

Feelings of dread, apprehension, or doom
Again, low blood sugar (hypoglycemia) or a low thyroid will cause these symptoms.

Difficulty concentrating, disorientation, mental confusion, memory lapses
These, too, are common symptoms of either low blood sugar (hypoglycemia) or a low thyroid

Hormone Replacement Therapy . . . .
When doctors talk about hormone replacement therapy (HRT), they are usually referring to a prescription for a combination of estradiol (conjugated estrogens) and synthetic progesterone. The

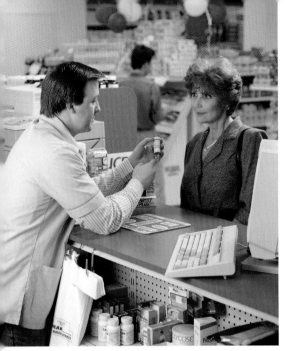

Conventional doctors rarely question the wisdom of multinational drug company marketing.

common prescription brands prescribed are Premarin®, an estrogen derived from the urine of pregnant mares, and Provera®, a chemically adulterated progesterone. There are still conventional doctors who only prescribe high doses of Premarin® (estrogen) without Provera® (progesterone), as well as another small group of doctors who believe that adding synthetic testosterone to the Premarin is an even better approach.

Doctors disagree about whether all menopausal women should be on hormones or whether hormones should be reserved for women with severe symptoms or those at high risk for bone loss and heart attacks. Some prescribe synthetic estrogen with or without progesterone to all their menopausal patients. Others, however, maintain that women should rarely be prescribed synthetic hormones and that symptoms can be controlled entirely by natural means. I fall into this latter category. However, sometimes HRT provides the only means by which some women can function as they would like.

Doctors also disagree about the length of time hormones should be taken. The extremist pharmaceutical view holds that menopausal women should be on hormones until death. Conventional doctors rarely question the wisdom of multinational drug company marketing. Conventional HRT is primarily supported by studies sponsored by the manufacturers of synthetic hormones. Despite the grandiose claims of this drug lobby, there is little scientific evidence to support the use of estrogen for the prevention of heart disease, osteoporosis or any other disease. Moreover, long-term studies on the effects of estrogen and progesterone on healthy postmenopausal women have never been done

Side Effects of Hormone Replacement Therapy

Conventional hormonal replacement therapy during menopause can cause:

Increased risk of breast cancer and uterine cancer
Both the breast and uterus can be stimulated to grow abnormally with estrogen supplementation. Supplementing with progesterone seems to reduce the risk of this happening but studies do indicate a greater risk of both cancers with the use of HRT.

Abnormal Pap tests
This is also due to the growth-stimulating effects of estrogen.

Abnormal bleeding with a resulting iron deficiency
This is caused by estrogen/progesterone imbalances, which are worsened by HRT.

Candida (yeast) infections
Estrogen stimulates fungal growth, whether the estrogen comes from the birth control pill or HRT.

Circulation problems
The estrogen in HRT can elevate blood pressure, cause a greater degree of blood clotting due to increased platelet stickiness, as well as depletion of vitamin B_6, leading to an increased risk of phlebitis, varicose veins and strokes.

Eye changes, pain, and visual disturbances
Estrogen causes changes in the cornea as well as in eye pressure, leading to visual disturbances.

High blood pressure
This is a direct result of too much estrogen, and it can cause strokes in susceptible women.

Abnormal blood clotting (thrombosis)
Estrogen causes changes in platelets and blood clotting factors, rendering them more sticky and likely to form clots (thrombosis).

Migraine
Neither the birth control pill nor HRT are recommended for those already suffering from migraines. In many cases, the migraines become worse.

Stroke
This is a consequence of high blood pressure and abnormal blood clotting, both caused by supplemented estrogen.

Increased risk of coronary artery disease
This is a consequence of high blood pressure and abnormal blood

clotting, both caused by supplemented estrogen. Studies also indicate that coronary artery disease increases when testosterone is deficient, a condition also made worse by conventional HRT. Since the average family doctor and gynecologist rarely measure hormone levels before, during, or after prescribing HRT, it is unlikely that low testosterone levels will be discovered in women who use HRT.

Weight gain
Estrogen increases fat deposition on the abdomen and hips.

Fluid retention
Estrogen increases fluid retention.

Loss of libido
This is due to inadequate progesterone relative to estrogen, or a testosterone deficiency, which is worsened by HRT.

Depression
Due to inadequate progesterone relative to estrogen.

Increase in breast lumps (fibrocystic breast disease)
Estrogen stimulates the growth of breast cysts.

Endometriosis
Estrogen stimulates the growth of endometrial tissue.

Diet for Menopausal Discomforts . . . .

Just about all the mental and physical discomforts of menopause can be successfully controlled by diet alone.

The standard Canadian or American diet is high in sugar and animal fats. Studies show that avoiding such foods and eating foods rich in soy protein can reduce both the frequency and the intensity of hot flashes, the most common menopause-related complaint. Soy contains plant hormones called phytoestrogens that act like weak estrogens but appear to be strong enough to prevent hot flashes and other menopausal discomforts. Japanese women who follow a traditional Japanese diet that includes soy products rarely need medical attention during their transition, and have virtually no incidence of osteoporosis.

The ideal diet for menopausal women is one that is closer to vegetarian, and is high in fiber and low in saturated fat and simple sugars. There are many reasons for this, the major one being that animal proteins, with their high phosphorus content, cause the body to lose large amounts of calcium and other minerals.

Red meat, chicken, and dairy products contain foreign estrogens and pesticide residues. Many other petrochemical compounds (xenoestrogens) with estrogenic properties are consumed in the food that is given to these animals, and they are subsequently concentrated in the milk and fat of the meat. These exogenous estrogens are then deposited in our fatty tissues and on estrogen and progesterone receptors where they are known to interfere in the proper utilization and production of progesterone and estrogen.

Eat as close to a natural diet as possible, cutting out all junk foods, soft drinks, processed foods, fried foods, white sugar, and other forms of refined carbohydrates. Avoid caffeine from sources such as coffee, tea, chocolate, and over-the-counter analgesics because caffeine intensifies menopausal discomforts. If you cannot become a complete vegetarian, replace red meat intake with cold-water fish like trout, salmon, cod, halibut, mackerel, and shark. Eat plenty of fresh fruits and vegetables, particularly dark leafy greens, as well as whole grains and legumes.

A high-fiber diet is important because of its beneficial effect on elimination. Whole psyllium seed husks, powdered flaxseed, guar gum, and bran have a binding effect on toxins in the colon, as well as harmful forms of estrogen metabolites and cholesterol, and are able to assist in the rapid excretion of these materials, thereby blocking their reabsorption into the bloodstream.

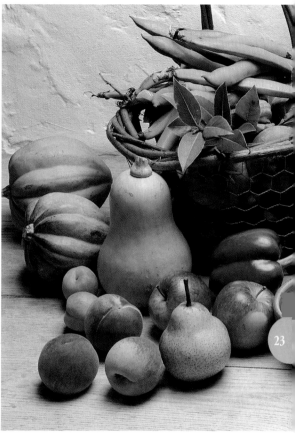

23

Eating a diet as close to nature as possible will help lessen or eliminate the mental and physical discomforts associated with menopause.

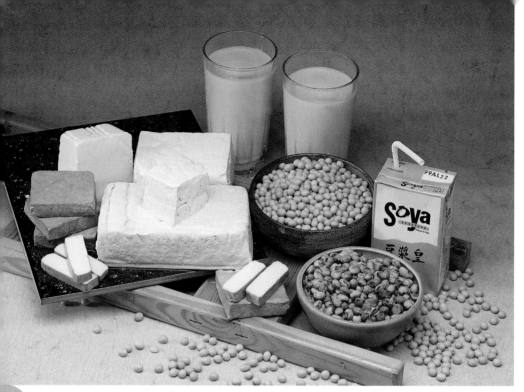

Eating foods rich in soy protein can reduce the frequency and intensity of hot flashes.

Phytoestrogens

To reverse menopausal problems with diet alone, a woman must be willing to consume more plants high in something called phytoestrogens. These compounds exert mild estrogenic effects through their content of isoflavones, phytosterols, saponins, or lignins.

Cultured soy products (organic, fermented) such as tofu, tempeh, and miso are high in genistein and other isoflavones known for their cholesterol-lowering effects as well as for their ability to prevent breast and prostate cancers. Substituting soy protein for animal protein a few times a day will decrease total cholesterol by as much as 10 percent, LDL cholesterol by 13 percent, and triglycerides by more than 10 percent, but without decreasing the "good" HDL cholesterol. One cup of soybeans will yield about 300 mg of isoflavones, the equivalent of 0.45 mg of prescription estrogens (1 tablet of conventional HRT).

There is some growing controversy about the use of large amounts of commercial soy products such as soymilk, infant soy formulas, and textured vegetable soy proteins (soy made to taste like chicken, pork, or turkey, etc.). These types of soy products should be consumed only occasionally. The high content of phytoestrogens in such processed foods has been causally linked to thyroid problems, infertility, and tumors, at least in experimental laboratory animals. Their adverse effects in humans are theoretical and remain to be proven. Be sure to buy fermented soy products only.

> ### Foods High in Phytoestrogens
> - Soy products (especially tofu, tempeh, and miso)
> - Fennel
> - Celery
> - Parsley
> - Clover sprouts
> - Milled (ground) flaxseed and flaxseed oil
> - Nuts and seeds
> - Corn oil

Nutritional Supplements for Menopause . . . . .

For women who can control hot flashes and other menopausal disturbances by diet alone, there is no great need to take any additional supplements. On the other hand, if dietary changes are ineffective or cannot be made for any number of reasons, nutritional supplements can provide convenient and very effective relief. The best documented of these are as follows:

Vitamin E will improve or reverse virtually all of the unpleasant menopausal symptoms as soon as one week after starting supplementation. Vitamin E has a documented benefit in reducing the risk of heart disease, cancer and other diseases caused by aging or low hormone levels. Suggested dosage: 200 to 800 IU daily.

Boron both enhances and mimics some of the effects of estrogen in postmenopausal women. Boron is also one of the most important minerals for healthy joints: a deficiency increases the risk of developing osteoarthritis. Boron is non-toxic, and supplementation with this mineral does not pose the same cancer-causing risks as synthetic estrogen replacement therapy. Suggested dosage: 3 to 6 mg daily

Essential fatty acids, found in hempseed oil capsules or a combination of flaxseed oil, evening primrose oil, and fish oils, provide high amounts of the omega-3, -6 and -9 essential fatty acids. The basic effect of these fats is to decrease the proinflammatory prostaglandin group of hormones while boosting the

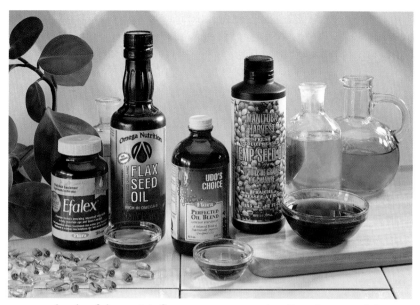

Essential fatty acids boost general health and lessen discomforts of menopause.

levels of the anti-inflammatory prostaglandins. Suggested dosage: 9,000 to 12,000 mg daily (eg. 1 tablespoon of flax oil plus six capsules of evening primrose oil).

> **Essential Fatty Acids**
> Essential fatty acids are called "essential" because we need them to survive, but the body does not make them itself. These fats are needed for a number of functions in the body and are necessary for energy production, brain function, healing, learning, athletic performance, beauty, and weight loss.

Bioflavonoids (hesperidin, catechin, rutin, quercetin, pycnogenols) work with vitamin C to maintain the integrity of the walls of capillaries and other blood vessels. They can, therefore, prevent excessive bleeding at any time in a woman's life, as well as hot flashes during menopause. Bioflavonoids are plant substances that exist together with vitamin C in nature. They prevent estrogens from being broken down too rapidly in the body, thereby ameliorating some unpleasant menopausal symptoms. Bioflavonoids are abundantly available in citrus fruits, garlic, onions, peppers, cherries, currants and buckwheat. Suggested dosage: 300 to 1,000 mg daily of bioflavonoids, and 1,000 mg or more daily of Vitamin C.

Vitamin A is helpful for women suffering from menorrhagia (excessive menstrual bleeding) during menopause. High doses of vitamin A stimulate a 100 percent greater production of estrogen in menopausal woman. In many cases hysterectomy can be avoided, and anemia due to excessive blood loss can be prevented. Suggested dosage: 25,000 IU twice daily.

Gamma-oryzanol is an antioxidant compound derived from rice bran oil that has been reported to relieve all menopausal discomforts in up to 85 percent of women who use the supplement for two months or longer–without side effects. While freely available from any health food store in the US gamma-oryzanol is difficult to find in Canada due to the suppressive regulations curtailing the availability of safe and effective nutritional supplements. Suggested dosage: 100 mg three times daily.

L-Tryptophan is an amino acid that is particularly effective against hot flashes, insomnia, and depression. L-Tryptophan is available in Canada only through a doctor's prescription. Suggested dosage: 1,000 to 6,000 mg daily.

Bee pollen is well known for its ability to provide energy. It contains nearly all of the B-complex vitamins, as well as folic acid, carotenoids, bioflavonoids, a wide variety of minerals and trace elements, essential fatty acids, and vitamins C, A, and E. Suggested dosage: 1 to 3 tsp (or 3 to 6 capsules) daily.

Royal jelly is another bee product with benefits for menopausal women. It contains small amounts of natural female hormones, minerals, B vitamins, folic acid, fatty acids, acetylcholine, amino acids, proteins, lipids, and carbohydrates. Royal jelly can help with the menopausal symptoms of chronic fatigue and low libido. Suggested dosage: 1 to 3 capsules three times daily.

Ipriflavone is derived from soy and occurs naturally in bee propolis. When taken with calcium it can restore bone density and prevent fractures in those with established osteoporosis. Ipriflavone has a chemical structure similar to that of estrogen but has no estrogenic or other hormonal activity. It can bind to estrogen receptors in bone tissue without exhibiting undesirable estrogenic effects on the breast and uterus. Ipriflavone may therefore be a safer alternative for many women, especially those predisposed to female cancers. Suggested dosage: 200 mg three times daily.

Velvet elk antler contains numerous compounds that are precursors to testosterone. Women with low libido caused by low testosterone levels who would rather not take prescription hormones usually find velvet elk antler very effective. Velvet elk antler has been used as a nutritional supplement in China for over 2,000 years, and is harvested humanely from specially bred elk during the rapid growth phase of antler development. Suggested dosage: 1 to 3 capsules daily.

Herbal Relief for Menopause . . . .

Some natural health care practitioners would opt to recommend herbs instead of nutritional supplements to support women through menopause. And there is now a growing body of medical evidence to add to the folklore supporting the use of certain popular herbs. The following is a list of the best documented of these remedies:

Black cohosh (*Cimicifuga racemosa*) exerts its benefits in menopause due to its estrogenic effects. Black cohosh extract is estriol-like in its behavior, making it a safe supplement for women with a high risk for breast and uterine cancers. No studies have ever reported side effects with black cohosh extract. Studies have shown that black cohosh, unlike synthetic estrogens (mainly variations of estradiol), does not produce endometrial thickening or tumors.

Black cohosh extract is the most widely used herbal approach to menopause. In Germany, Scandinavia, and Austria it is the number one remedy for menopausal discomforts. I usually recommend that women using this herb stop taking it from time to time to see if menopausal problems return. Some women will experience no return of menopausal problems after stopping black cohosh extract after six months; others might see

> There is a growing body of medical evidence to add to the folklore supporting the use of certain popular herbs to ease discomforts brought on by menopause.

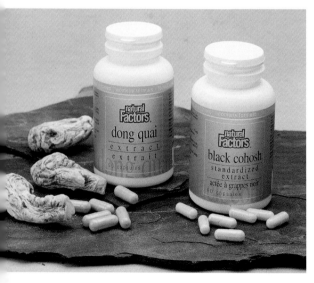

a return of symptoms. In any case, black cohosh is safe to take for years on end. Suggested dosage: 1 to 2 tablets twice daily of the standardized 27-deoxyacteine herbal extract.

Dong quai (*Angelica sinensis*) is helpful for any menopausal discomfort. Like black cohosh extract, dong quai has mild estrogenic (estriol-like) effects, as well as the ability to stabilize blood vessels. This herb also has a very good reputation as an effective treatment for a number of female conditions, including premenstrual syndrome treatment and painful menses (dysmenorrhea). Suggested dosage: 1 to 2 capsules three or four times daily when needed.

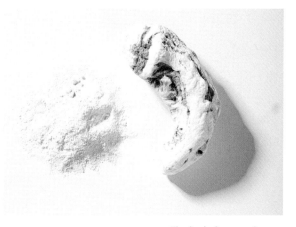

The herb dong quai is helpful for any menopausal discomfort because of its mild estrogenic effects.

Licorice (*Glycyrrhiza glabra*) is helpful for menopausal problems of any kind. Like black cohosh and dong quai, licorice root has mild estrogenic (estriol-like) activity. It also has the ability to protect adrenal hormones (DHEA, cortisol) from being broken down too rapidly by the body, resulting in a net increase in the body's adrenal hormone levels. One should exercise some caution in using licorice as blood pressure could become elevated due to the increase of adrenal steroids. Suggested dosage: 1 to 2 capsules three or four times daily when needed.

Panax ginseng (Chinese or Korean ginseng), usually thought to be a good male tonic, also has estrogenic (estriol-like) activity. Panax ginseng is used as a general tonic and has a number of health-enhancing properties, such as its ability to improve psychological function in postmenopausal women. Some women find it effective for hot flashes, low energy, low sex drive, and mental fogginess. Panax ginseng saponins stimulate corticosteroid production, making it an extremely useful remedy in women where the majority of the menopausal symptoms are caused by severe stress and weak adrenal glands. Studies also indicate that it enhances the ability of licorice to increase serum cortisol concentrations.

High doses can be a problem: some women have reported postmenopausal bleeding with particularly potent versions of this supplement. Panax ginseng can also be too stimulating for some people, causing symptoms like transiently high blood pressure, palpitations, and anxiety–all of which are reversible with the discontinuation of the supplement. Not all ginsengs on the market are created equally. The contents of preparations labeled as containing Panax ginseng can vary greatly from brand to brand in their content of the active ingredients (the ginsenosides). Check with an herbalist or read labels carefully in choosing an effective supplement. Suggested dosage: 1 to 3 capsules daily of a standardized ginsenoside extract.

Chaste berry (*Vitex agnus castus*) is another very beneficial menopausal remedy. This herb appears to work by stimulating the pituitary gland to manufacture more progesterone and less estrogen. However, it also inhibits androgens (the male hormones) and can, therefore, reduce sex drive. Suggested dosage: 1 to 3 capsules daily.

Unicorn root (*Aletris farinosa*), like wild yam, contains diosgenin and has some mild hormonal activity. Seldom used on its own, this herb is most often seen as one of the many components in multi-herbal capsules designed for helping with menopausal discomforts. Suggested dosage: 1 to 3 capsules daily.

Many natural health practitioners recommend herbs to treat the side effects of menopause.

David Jennings

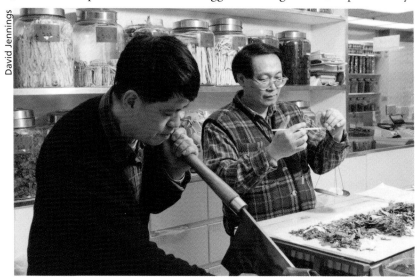

Sarsaparilla (*Smilax*) may help some menopausal women with joint problems. Sarsaparilla can have antirheumatic, antiseptic, and antipruritic (anti-itch) activity. Although used by both men and women to boost athletic performance, the sterols contained in sarsaparilla are not anabolic steroids nor are they converted in the body to anabolic steroids. And contrary to popular belief, testosterone has never been detected in any plant, including sarsaparilla. Suggested dosage: 1 to 3 capsules daily.

Most women require the use of only one of these herbal supplements, but some may need to use a combination of two or even three herbs. It all depends on biochemical individuality. My advice is to try the black cohosh extract first. It should work favorably 85 to 90 percent of the time. If you need to add another herb for better control of hot flashes or other discomforts, go with dong quai, then licorice, and on down the list. If no combination of these herbs works for you then you are one of those rare women who need to consider using natural progesterone cream or one of the other natural hormones discussed in the next section.

Natural Hormone Replacement Therapy . . . . .

The only real natural hormone replacement therapy (NHRT) is that provided by diet, and nutritional and herbal supplements. For the most part, these can be obtained in either the grocery store or the health food store. Beyond this, what we are really dealing with is drugs. Natural progesterone in a wild yam base comes from a drug company, not from the wild yam.

Wild Yam Cream

Wild yam cream is often touted as a natural source of progesterone, and, therefore, as an effective treatment for menopausal symptoms. Mexican wild yam (*Dioscorea*) is effective as a treatment for some menstrual irregularities but does not appear to be effective for menopausal problems. Its claim to fame, however, is that its active ingredient, diosgenin, is used by pharmaceutical companies to manufacture a variety of steroid hormones, including progesterone, testosterone, DHEA, and the estrogens. Wild yam creams do not naturally contain progesterone, as is mistakenly thought by those who are strong believers in the use of natural progesterone creams for menopause. If a wild yam cream contains progesterone it is only because the molecules naturally present in the wild yam have been chemically changed into progesterone, which is then added to a cream.

Many doctors, including holistic medical doctor Jonathan Wright (who devoted an entire book to the subject recently (see *Natural Hormone Replacement*, Smart Publications, 1997), are of the opinion that the use of natural progesterone, as well as estriol, estradiol, estrone, testosterone, and DHEA is natural hormone replacement therapy. Technically it is not.

To get such products in Canada they must be compounded by a pharmacist under a medical doctor's prescription. In addition, the raw ingredients that make up these prescriptions, although purportedly identical to what the body produces, are manufactured in a laboratory and sold to pharmacists by drug companies. In both Canada and the US, "natural" hormones are under the control of multinational drug companies. You cannot use them on your own but must consult with a doctor.

Once again, I have to stress that it is the rare menopausal woman that needs this sort of therapy. While considered safer than conventional forms of HRT, the jury is still out on the safety of broad-scale use of these pharmaceuticals. Compared to herbal remedies–which have been used for centuries without significant incident–the quasi-natural therapies advocated by more and more medical doctors have not withstood the test of time with respect to long-term safety.

Nevertheless, if you believe in NHRT I would recommend that before supplementing any of these hormonal remedies you have lab tests done to verify hormonal levels. Research now shows that saliva testing is more accurate than blood tests for assessing the levels of these and other hormones.

Saliva testing is more accurate than the blood tests because steroid hormones like DHEA are carried around the bloodstream complexed with a carrier protein. The active hormone is "free," meaning that it does not have a protein carrier. Blood tests do not distinguish between the free and the bound form of the hormone while the saliva test only measures the free (active) hormone and is therefore a more accurate reflection of that hormone's activity.

Some labs in the US offer saliva testing directly to the public, thereby avoiding the necessity of consulting a doctor. (See "Sources" for further information.) If you feel more comfortable working with a doctor, saliva hormone testing can also be ordered and interpreted for you by your doctor.

While DHEA, natural progesterone, and other natural hormones are readily available in the US without a prescription, in Canada, a doctor's prescription is necessary. The tests, however, are available to anyone without a doctor's approval and are a good first step toward optimizing your hormone levels.

The Hormones Replaced
Estrogens

The healthy adult woman makes three different estrogens in her ovaries: estrone (10 to 20 percent), estradiol (10 to 20 percent) and estriol (60 to 80 percent). Most conventional HRT is close to 100 percent estradiol, and it is this estrogen that is considered to increase the growth of breast and uterine tissue, thus increasing the risk of breast and uterine cancers.

Estriol, on the other hand, prevents these cancers, and is the favored hormone in NHRT. Natural estrogens (in a ratio of 8:1:1 estriol:estradiol:estrone) can be used in oral capsule form to be swallowed once daily, or as a cream applied to the body. The hormones in the cream are absorbed through the skin and enter the bloodstream in this manner. If one uses estrogen in NHRT, it must still be balanced by progesterone in order to prevent something called estrogen dominance.

Estrogen Dominance

Under the normal, healthy circumstances of a woman's monthly cycle, estrogen is the dominant hormone for the first two weeks and is balanced by progesterone, which is the dominant hormone for the latter two weeks. When progesterone levels fail to reach the normal 20 to 25 mg during the final two weeks of a woman's monthly cycle then estrogen is unopposed for the entire month. This condition is referred to as "estrogen dominance."

If the estrogen percent becomes higher than the normal ratio to progesterone, many women start to show the following symptoms:

- Breast tenderness
- Decreased sex drive
- Depression
- Endometriosis
- Fibrocystic breasts
- Headaches and migraines
- High blood pressure (hypertension)
- Memory loss/Foggy thinking
- Osteoporosis
- Uterine fibroids
- Water retention and swelling
- Weight gain

Progesterone

Progesterone is made in the body from cholesterol. It is the precursor for many hormones, including estrogen, cortisol, and testosterone. It also promotes a more efficient use of thyroid hormone by the body. Aside from its role in reversing osteoporosis, progesterone protects against breast cancer, decreases fibrocystic breast disease and reduces the incidence of ovarian cysts. It prevents fluid retention, fat deposits, vaginal dryness, and urinary bladder infections. Women who suffer from both stress and a loss of libido will benefit from progesterone supplementation. For more information on the use of natural progesterone, see Dr. John Lee's book, *What Your Doctor May Not Tell You About Menopause* (Warner Books, 1996).

Natural hormone replacement therapy involves the use of natural progesterone cream and combinations of progesterone with natural estriol, estradiol, estrone, and testosterone. For many natural health care practitioners, progesterone cream is the single most important supplement for menopausal symptoms.

Oral progesterone is not as effective as the natural progesterone cream. The cream absorbs through the skin and goes directly to where it is needed by the body. The transdermal route ensures that the progesterone bypasses the liver for more efficient delivery to receptor sites. It can be applied once daily into soft tissue areas such as the chest, breast, under arms, inner thighs or abdomen. The total *monthly* dosage is 1,000 mg (equivalent to approximately one-half tsp of cream daily). There are usually no side effects, but some sensitive women may experience a temporary increase in menstrual bleeding as well as hot

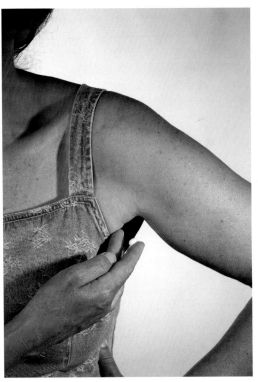

Natural progesterone cream can be applied to soft tissue areas of the body, such as under the arms, where it absorbs through the skin.

flashes, since progesterone has a thermogenic (temperature elevating) effect. Remember that progesterone is produced naturally by the body at levels as high as 400 mg daily during pregnancy: natural progesterone cream delivers between 15 and 20 mg of progesterone daily.

Do not confuse natural progesterone cream with "progestins" or "progestagens." These are different forms of synthetic progesterone that are only available by prescription, and they are associated with many significant side effects. With natural progesterone cream, the body uses only what it needs and no excess is allowed to build up. Natural progesterone is initially absorbed into the body's fat tissues, and it takes about three or four months before blood levels increase significantly. However, the benefits of progesterone cream may be seen much earlier.

Progesterone and Osteoporosis

Synthetic estrogens in pill or cream form may increase the risk for breast and uterine cancer and, moreover, have virtually no impact on an already osteoporotic skeleton. Yes, estrogens slow down osteoporosis. They do not, however, reverse it like natural progesterone. Studies done by gynecologists, internists, and other types of doctors conclude that progesterone is far more important than estrogen in both the prevention and treatment of osteoporosis. Aside from its role in reversing osteoporosis, progesterone cream protects against breast cancer, decreases fibrocystic breast disease, and reduces the incidence of ovarian cysts. It prevents fluid retention, fat deposits, vaginal dryness, and urinary bladder infections. Women who suffer from both stress and a loss of libido will also benefit from the use of progesterone cream.

The wild yam cream that is sold in health food stores does not contain any progesterone. It may have some value as a natural moisturizer but will do virtually nothing for menopausal discomforts. Contrary to popular belief there is no conversion to progesterone upon application and absorption through the skin. Only a synthetic process is capable of converting compounds in wild yam cream into progesterone. The body simply cannot do it.

Due to some peculiar politics, and not for any specific health reasons, natural progesterone cream can no longer be sold in health food stores in Canada. For the time being, if you are Canadian, your only alternatives are the health food stores in the US, or a prescription for the progesterone cream from your doctor, which is then purchased from a pharmacy that employs a compounding pharmacist. In the latter situation, the pharmacist makes up the progesterone cream from raw ingredients, including natural progesterone. The usual progesterone content of such creams is 3 percent, but 6 percent or higher potencies can be made up for individualized needs.

DHEA (dehydroepiandrosterone)

It was once thought that DHEA was merely a precursor to other hormones like testosterone and estrogen, and that it had no other specific role of its own. Studies done on both animals and humans in the past decade, however, have shown that this is not true. In fact, epidemiological studies show that higher DHEA levels are associated with increased longevity, less cancer and less heart disease, thus suggesting that at least some aging manifestations may be caused by DHEA deficiency. It has also been shown that DHEA blood levels decline progressively with age, a phenomenon that does not occur with any other adrenal steroid.

DHEA is available in health food stores in the US without a doctor's prescription. In Canada, the Health Protection Branch banned the sale of DHEA in November 1996, raising the ire of thousands of people across Canada. The banning of DHEA has been mistakenly interpreted by some to suggest that it is in some way toxic or harmful. It is not, and there is no evidence to suggest that DHEA is any more harmful than the birth control pill (a steroid) or over-the-counter cortisone (steroid) creams.

Many published studies support the use of supplemental DHEA during menopause, especially as a treatment for osteoporosis and low libido.

While it is true that the long-term effects of daily DHEA supplementation are not fully known, the same can be said for many of the prescription and non-prescription drugs given quick approval without long-term safety and efficacy studies. The concerns expressed about long-term use of DHEA relate to its potential ability to increase the risk of breast and prostate cancers. Neither of these two possibilities has been proven by any studies and, to date, these concerns remain speculative.

DHEA is generally considered to be safe for short-term use. Until more is known about its long-term effects, DHEA should be used with caution and with the supervision of a health care practitioner.

Testosterone

Menopausal women are sometimes prescribed testosterone, the major male hormone. Both men and women manufacture testosterone, which has a profound effect on libido as well as the heart, cholesterol levels, muscle strength and bone density. Low levels of testosterone are comon in menopausal women.

Testosterone is anabolic, which means that it helps to build protein tissue, including muscles, bones and connective tissue like ligaments, cartilage, and tendons. It has an important role in preventing osteoporosis in both men and women.

Testosterone, unfortunately, has been tainted with a bad reputation due to the many weight lifters and athletes who misuse the synthetic analogues of man made testosterone, called anabolic steroids.

The taking of excessive doses of anabolic steroids can result in serious adverse consequences such as liver damage and perhaps even some forms of cancer. On the other hand, a deficiency of testosterone can cause a weakness in muscles and bones as well as in numerous other tissues and organs.

Testosterone also helps regulate the immune system. People with autoimmune disorders (rheumatoid arthritis, systemic lupus erythematosus, multiple sclerosis) all appear to benefit from

37

Low levels of testosterone, the major male hormone, are common in menopausal women.

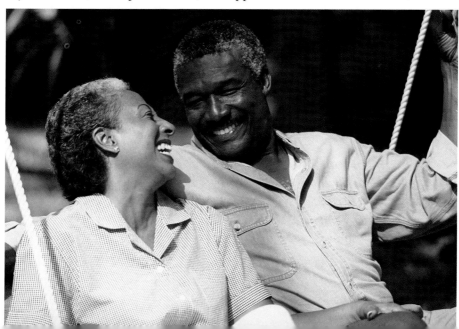

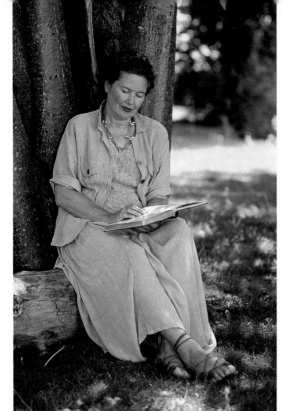

Only you can choose to take control of the natural transition known as menopause.

testosterone therapy. Due to its ability to optimize blood sugar levels, testosterone therapy can improve appetite, increase weight in underweight individuals, improve wound healing and increase resistance to infection. Although testosterone builds body mass by helping the body create larger muscles, it simultaneously gets rid of excess fat and reduces obesity.

Testosterone lowers serum cholesterol and triglycerides and has been used in Europe to treat patients with circulatory problems like gangrene of the feet, coronary artery heart disease, high blood pressure and other cardiovascular diseases. Positive attitudes, general motivation, aggression, and sex drive all seem to be related to tissue levels of testosterone.

In women, the major side effect of the use of testosterone is excessive facial hair growth, acne, and male pattern baldness.

Androstenedione

Androstenedione is a male hormone produced in the gonads and adrenal glands of both men and women from either DHEA or progesterone. It is a direct precursor and metabolite of testosterone. In the body, androstenedione and testosterone convert back and forth to each other depending on the need by the body for one or the other hormone. In women who have lost the functioning of their ovaries due to disease, surgery or menopause, androstenedione becomes the major source of estrogen production. With menopause, progesterone levels fall and the body responds to this by increasing its production of androstenedione.

Androstenedione supplementation increases testosterone production and enhances libido almost immediately. German studies have shown up to a 237 percent increase in free testosterone levels after a 100 mg dose of androstenedione. Free testosterone levels may begin rising in as little as fifteen minutes after taking androstenedione on an empty stomach.

One of the problems with androstenedione is that it will also eventually convert to estrogen; thus estrogen levels can go excessively high, worsening estrogen dominance problems. Another problem for most women is that the higher levels of testosterone can lead to undesirable side effects like male pattern hair loss. For this reason, it is better to use natural remedies without these potential side effects. Alternatively, if the natural products do not enhance a woman's libido during menopause, the use of this hormone on a once-a-week basis (50 to 100 mg once weekly) may be just enough to produce the desired result without significant masculinization.

Pregnenelone

Pregnenelone is a made in the body from cholesterol and then converted into DHEA, primarily in the adrenal glands. It is also produced to some degree in the ovaries, liver, brain and the testes. Pregnenelone is also a precursor to estrogen, testosterone, progesterone, and DHEA. Known as the "feel good" hormone, pregneneolone has been used successfully for balancing adrenal and ovarian hormones, improving poor memory, fatigue, stress, and PMS. Pregnenolone is far less likely to cause masculinizing side effects than both DHEA and androstenedione.

Supplements of pregnenolone became available over the counter in 1995 in the US. In Canada, however, one needs a doctor's prescription to get it.

Take Control of Your Transition . . . .

Menopause need not be suppressed, drugged, or stopped. Only you can choose to take control of this natural transition in your life. Knowledge of the facts and the options open to you give you the power and control to take your health into your own hands. It is your perception—not that of the media, doctor or drug company—that is important. I wish you good health and a natural transition.

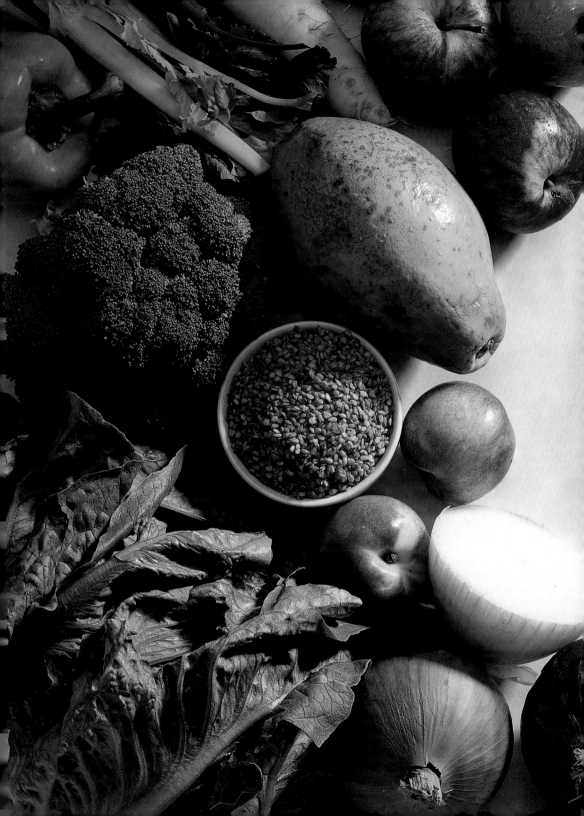

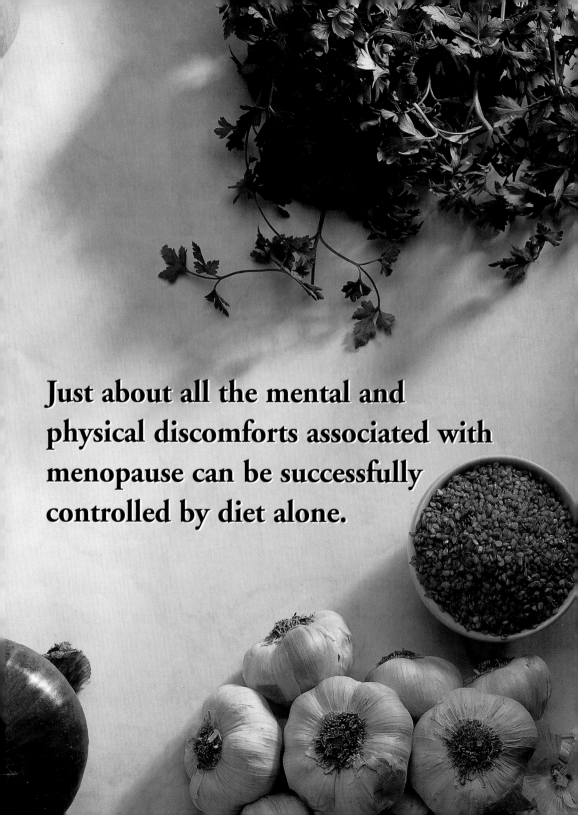

Just about all the mental and physical discomforts associated with menopause can be successfully controlled by diet alone.

Waffles with Fruit and Kamut Cereal

Eat fruit raw whenever possible to preserve enzymes and other heat-sensitive nutrients like vitamin C and calcium. Eating calcium-rich foods is important during menopause as calcium absorption is decreased in the early phases.

Waffles:

1 ½ cups (375 ml) **chickpea flour**

2 tsp **baking powder**

½ tsp **sea salt**

2 tsp **natural sugar crystals**

2 large **free-range eggs, yolks separated**

1 cup (250 ml) **rice milk**

⅓ cup (80 ml) **butter, melted**

Fruit and Cereal:

1 cup (250 ml) **strawberries**

1 cup (250 ml) **watermelon, sliced**

1 cup (250 ml) **grapes, sliced**

1 cup (250 ml) **mango, sliced**

1 cup (250 ml) **pear, sliced**

1 cup (250 ml) **apple, sliced**

2 cups (500 ml) **kamut flakes**

¼ cup (60 ml) **almond slivers**

1 cup (250 ml) **rice milk**

To prepare the waffles, sift flour, baking powder, and salt into a medium bowl. Stir in sugar.

In another bowl, beat together egg yolks, rice milk, and melted butter. Add to dry ingredients and beat thoroughly. In another bowl, beat egg whites until stiff then fold into batter.

Heat waffle iron, but do not grease. (To test for correct heat, put 1 teaspoon of water inside waffle iron, close and heat until steaming stops.) Spoon 1 tablespoon of batter into the center of each compartment. Close and cook until puffed and golden brown then lift waffle out with a fork.

Arrange fruit onto plates. Place kamut in bowls, add almonds and pour rice milk over top. Serve with the waffles.

Yields 6 waffles

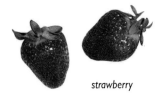

strawberry

Natural Sugar

Natural sugar crystals may be equally substituted for the white sugar called in your recipes. There are many types of natural sugar crystals on the market. Some are superior to others simply because of the way they're made. I use either Sucanat or Rapadura, which is dried cane juice and totally unrefined. Unlike the process used to make white refined sugar, the process used to make these natural sugars preserves the natural rich flavor and nutrition, without preservatives or additives, and actually results in a lower level of sucrose than refined sugar.

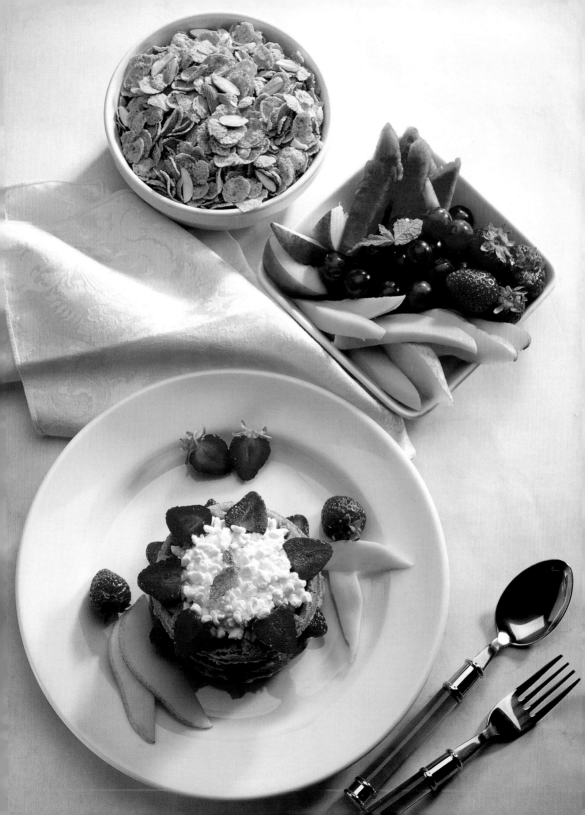

Avocado-Tomato Salad with Frisée

The avocado in this delicious salad supplies the vitamin E you need to regulate estrogen levels, while the frisée lettuce (also called curly endive or chicory) and tomatoes are full of vitamin C to help the vitamin E work properly.

1 ripe avocado, cut in ½" (1 cm) chunks

1 large ripe tomato, cut in ½" (1 cm) chunks

1 small white onion, cut in ½" (1 cm) chunks

4 cloves garlic, roasted

2 cups (300 g) frisée lettuce

Dressing:

2 tbsp apple cider vinegar

2 tbsp cold-pressed flax seed oil

1 tbsp fresh lemon juice

1 tbsp extra-virgin olive oil

1 tsp ginger, minced

Pinch mustard powder

Sea salt and freshly ground pepper, to taste

In a large bowl, whisk together all the dressing ingredients. Gently toss the avocado, tomato, onion, and garlic with half the dressing. Place onto plates, arrange frisée lettuce over top and drizzle with remaining dressing.

Serves 2

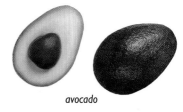

avocado

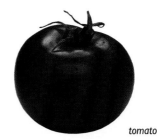

tomato

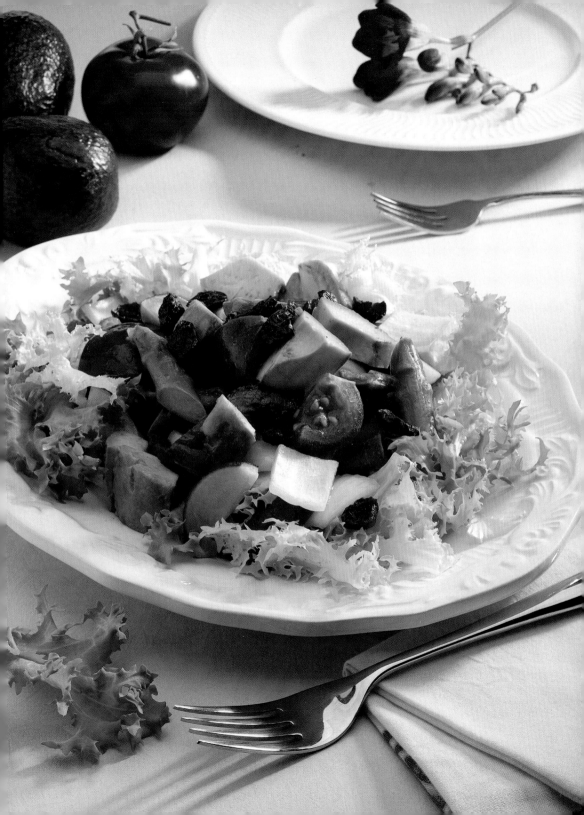

Marinated Mushrooms with Salsa

Green leafy vegetables provide enzymes and vitamins as well as a good dietary source of calcium.

4 Shiitake or Maitake mushrooms, or 2 large Portobello mushrooms

2 tbsp extra-virgin olive oil

2 large radicchio leaves

2 cups (250 g) mixed greens

Marinade:

2 tbsp extra-virgin olive oil

1 tbsp freshly squeezed lemon juice

½ tsp dried rosemary or 1 tsp fresh rosemary, chopped

Sea salt and freshly ground pepper, to taste

Salsa:

½ cup (125 g) cucumber, diced

½ cup (125 g) each red and yellow bell pepper, diced

½ cup (125 g) green onion, chopped

1 tbsp fresh cilantro, chopped

1 clove garlic, minced

2 tbsp cold-pressed olive oil or flax seed oil

Clean the mushrooms with a pastry brush or towel (do not wash them, since mushrooms, especially Portobello, absorb a lot of water). Remove the stems and scrape out the inside black parts with a spoon.

In a bowl, whisk together the marinade ingredients. Add mushrooms and let sit for ½ hour to 2 hours.

In a medium-size bowl, combine all the salsa ingredients. Refrigerate.

In a frying pan, heat oil over medium heat and sauté mushrooms until soft.

Arrange 1 radicchio leaf in the shape of a cup onto each plate. Place mushroom into the radicchio cups and arrange mixed greens around. Serve with the salsa.

Serves 2

red bell pepper

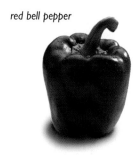

1 tbsp apple cider vinegar

Juice of ½ lemon

Sea salt and freshly ground pepper, to taste

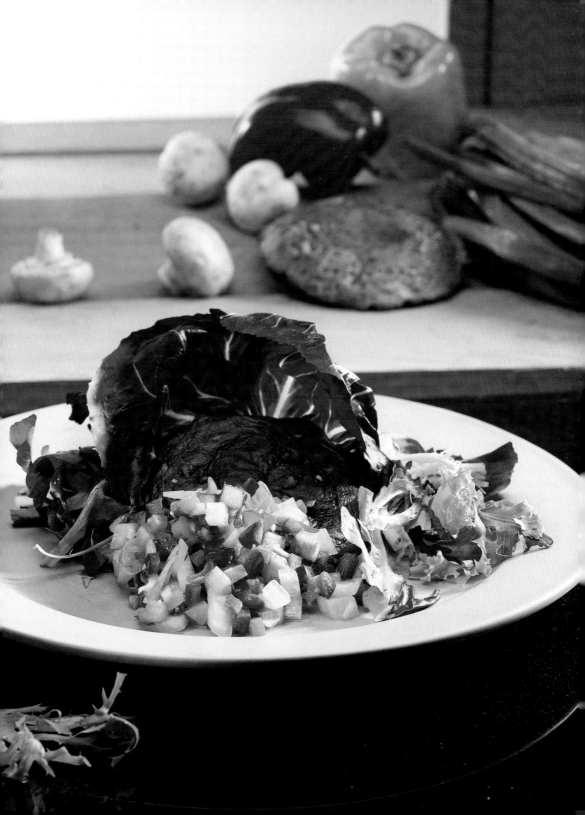

Sprout Chickpea Salad

Alfalfa sprouts provide high amounts of minerals, protein, and vitamins A, B complex, C, D, E, and K. Clover sprouts are high in phytoestrogens. The B vitamins are important for healthy liver function needed to detoxify excess hormones.

1 ½ cups (300 g) **clover or alfalfa sprouts**

1 cup (250 g) **cooked chickpeas**

2 cups (240 g) **endive leaves**

4-6 baby carrots, peeled

2 large ripe tomatoes, cut in wedges

1 small cucumber, sliced

1 cup (250 g) **mushrooms, sliced**

Dressing:

4 tbsp cold-pressed walnut or flax seed oil

2 tbsp freshly squeezed lemon juice

2 tbsp apple cider vinegar

1 tsp Dijon mustard

Sea salt and freshly ground pepper, to taste

1 tsp fresh thyme, chopped

In a bowl, whisk together all dressing ingredients. Arrange the vegetables, chickpeas, and mushroom onto plates and drizzle with dressing. (Do not toss this salad, since sprouts are very delicate.)

Serves 2

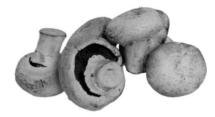

mushrooms

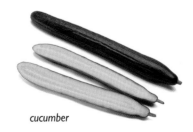

cucumber

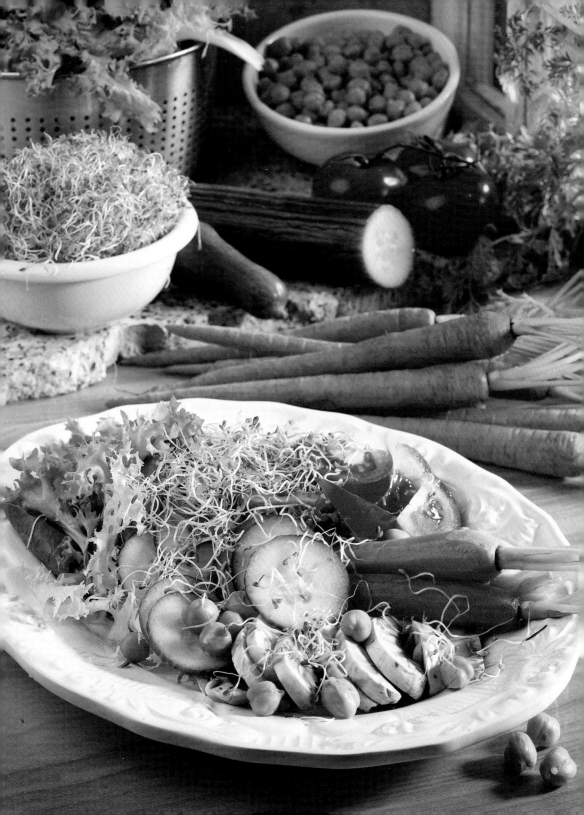

Tomato-Fennel Soup

The versatile tomato is an excellent source of vitamin C and a good source of vitamins E and B complex, important vitamins for hormone regulation and reducing stress.

2 cups (500 ml) **fennel, chopped**

1 cup (250 ml) **celery, chopped**

1 small white onion, chopped

3 cloves garlic, minced

2 tbsp extra-virgin olive oil

3 cups (750 ml) **tomatoes, chopped**

2 cups (500 ml) **vegetable stock**

1 bay leaf

Sea salt and freshly ground pepper, to taste

¼ cup (60 ml) **green onion, for garnish**

Fennel leaves, for garnish

In a large pot, heat oil over medium heat and sauté fennel, celery, onion, and garlic until tender. Add tomato, vegetable stock, bay leaf and season with salt and pepper. Cover and simmer for 5 to 7 minutes.

Remove the bay leaf then pour the soup into a food processor or blender and purée until smooth. Return to the pot, stir and heat through.

Pour the soup into bowls, garnish with green onions and sprigs of fennel leaves, and serve.

Serves 2

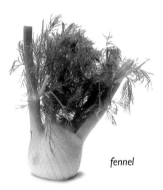

fennel

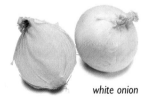

white onion

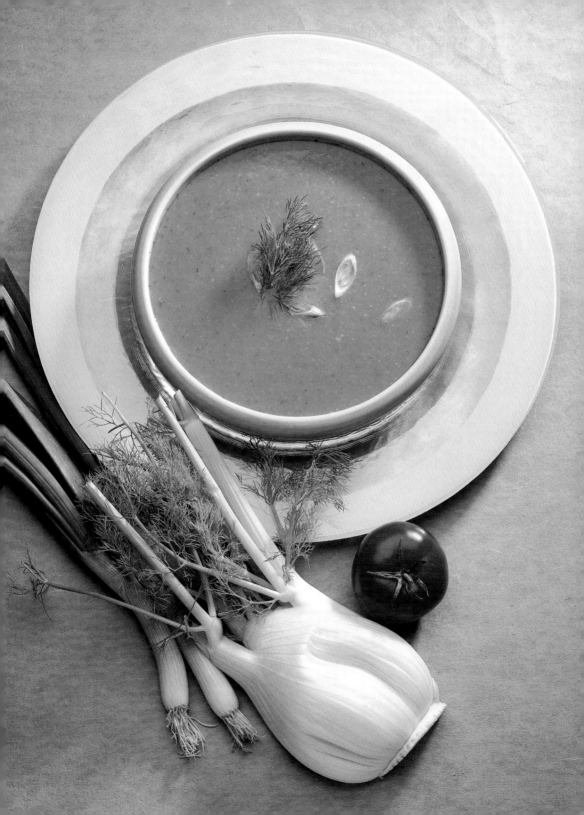

Shiitake Miso

Miso, a traditional Japanese staple, is an important food for treating menopause discomforts. Try the robust soy (hatcho) miso, which is grain-free and fermented longer than other types of miso.

1 cup (250 ml) **rice noodles**

1 cup (250 ml) **shiitake mushrooms, sliced**

1 clove garlic, minced

1 tbsp extra-virgin olive oil

2 cups (500 ml) **vegetable stock**

1 tbsp soy miso

¼ cup (60 ml) **green onions, sliced**

1 cup (250 ml) **soy bean sprouts**

1 tbsp red bell pepper, minced

Place rice noodles in a large bowl and pour salted boiling water over top. Soak for 7 to 10 minutes then drain and set aside.

In a pot, heat oil and sauté mushroom and garlic. Add vegetable stock and simmer for 3 to 4 minutes. Stir in rice noodles, miso, green onion, and sprouts. Garnish with bell pepper and serve immediately.

Serves 2

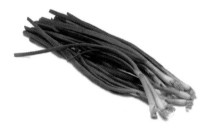

green onion

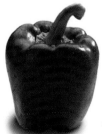

red pepper

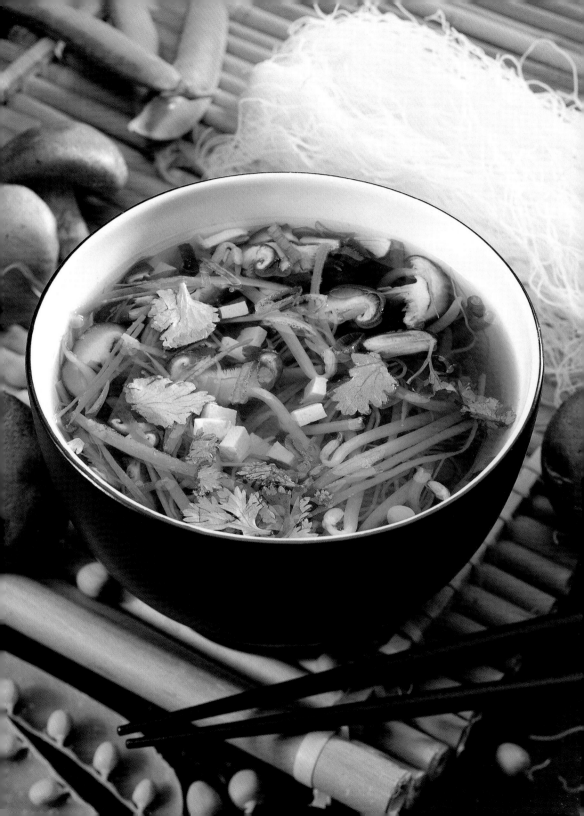

Pepper Trio with Tempeh

A delicious whole food made out of fermented soy beans, tempeh is highly digestible and protein-rich, and is also an important source of vitamin B12 for vegetarians.

1 cup (250 ml) **carrots, diced**

1 cup (250 ml) **celery, diced**

½ cup (125 ml) **onion, minced**

2 cloves garlic, minced

1 tbsp ginger, minced

2 tbsp extra-virgin olive oil

1 tbsp butter

1 ½ cups (375 ml) **short-grain brown rice, cooked**

1 tbsp cilantro, chopped

1 tbsp dill, chopped

1 block tempeh, cubed

½ cup (125 ml) **green peas**

Dash tamari

1 each red, yellow, and green bell peppers, cut in half

1 cup (250 ml) **soy bean sprouts, for garnish**

Sauce:

2 tbsp tamari

2 tbsp roasted sesame seed oil

1 ½ tbsp tahini

1 tsp fresh lime or lemon juice

In a pan, heat oil and butter over medium heat then saute carrot, celery, onion, garlic and ginger until tender. Stir in rice, tempeh, peas and herbs; season with a dash of tamari. Remove from heat and place about 2 tablespoons of the mixture into each pepper half. Place peppers into a bamboo steamer and steam for 5 to 7 minutes.

In the meantime, whisk sauce ingredients together in a bowl.

Place soy bean sprouts onto plates and arrange peppers over top. Drizzle with sauce and serve.

Serves 2

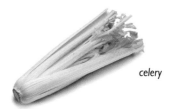

celery

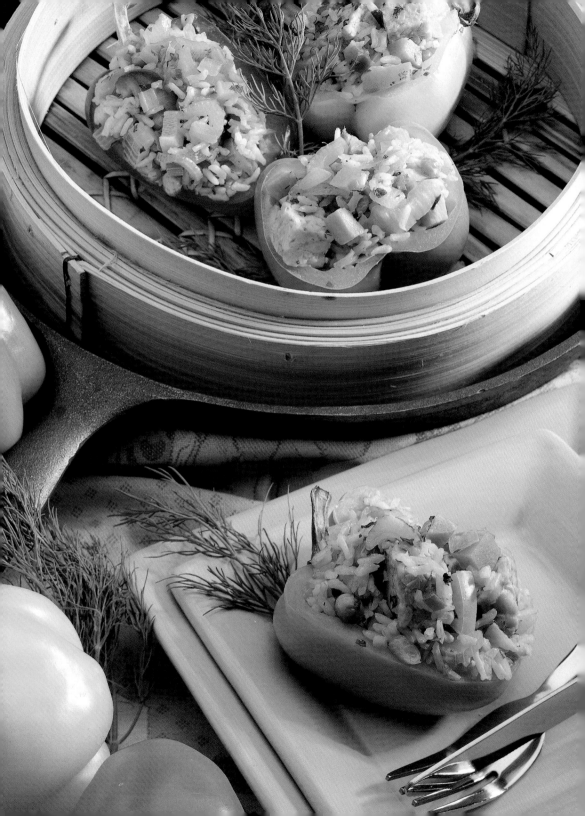

Kamut Risotto with Vegetable

This tangy fiber-rich dish warms and comforts, and by the way, also helps the body excrete harmful toxins and estrogen metabolites.

1 ½ cups (375 ml) **kamut risotto**

2 tbsp extra-virgin olive oil

2 cloves garlic, minced

½ cup (125 ml) **onion, diced**

1 tbsp ground turmeric

3 cups (750 ml) **water**

1 tbsp organic butter

½ cup (125 ml) **carrot, diced**

½ cup (125 ml) **red bell pepper, diced**

½ cup (125 ml) **yellow bell pepper, diced**

½ cup (125 ml) **green onions, chopped**

2 tbsp fresh rosemary, chopped

2 tbsp freshly squeezed lemon juice

In a pot, heat oil on medium heat and sauté risotto, garlic, onion, and turmeric until oil is fully absorbed. Add rosemary and water and cook until almost all the water is absorbed. Stir in butter, carrot, peppers, and season with salt and pepper. Cook for 4 to 6 minutes then stir in green onion and lemon juice and cook for 1 to 2 minutes longer.

Garnish with fresh rosemary sprigs and serve.

Serves 2

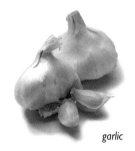

garlic

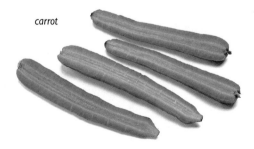

carrot

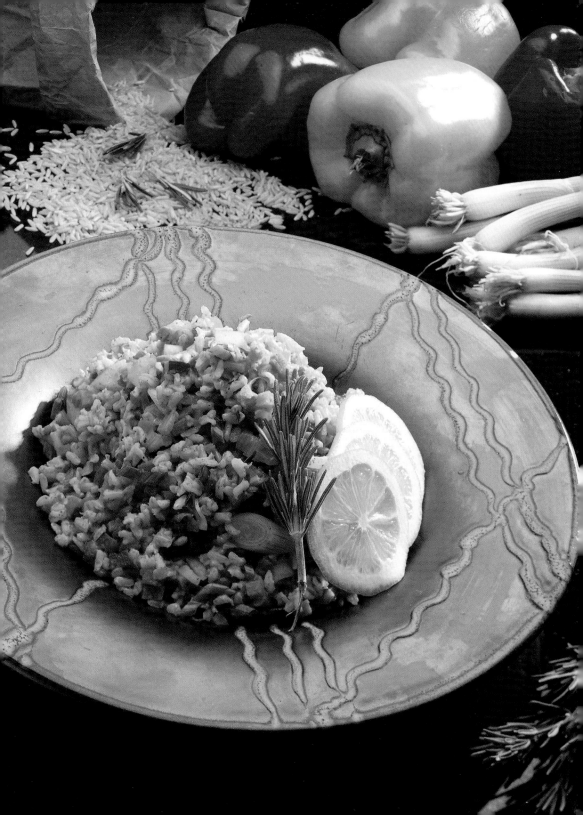

Salmon Filet on a Bed of Tabouhli

Tabouhli is a noodle type of couscous best served at room temperature. It is a good source of fiber and carbohydrates and tastes very refreshing especially during the hot summer. Lime juice gives a unique flavor and prevents your body from dehydrating.

Tahbouli:

1 cup (250 ml) **tabouhli**

1 ½ cups (375 ml) **water**

Pinch sea salt

1 cup (250 ml) **cucumber, diced**

1 cup (250 ml) **tomato, diced**

1 cup (250 ml) **bell pepper, diced**

1 cup (250 ml) **onion, diced**

1 clove garlic, minced

1 tbsp cilantro, chopped

1 tbsp parsley, chopped

2 tbsp extra-virgin olive oil

Juice of ½ lime

Salmon:

2 fresh sockeye or spring salmon filets (⅓ lb or 155 g each)

2 tbsp extra-virgin olive oil

Herbamare, to taste

Dash tamari

Rinse tabouhli and dry well. Cook in salted water for 7 to 10 minutes or until soft. In a bowl, combine oil, lime juice, garlic, cilantro, and parsley. Stir in all diced vegetables then add the tabouhli and mix well. Set aside at room temperature.

Bring a pot of salted water to a boil and blanch the carrots for 4 to 5 minutes. Drain and immediately rinse with cold water.

In a pan, heat oil over medium heat and panroast the salmon for 3 to 4 minutes each side, seasoning with Herbamare and dash of tamari. In the same pan, roast carrots and Belgian endive for 1 to 2 minutes each side until slightly warm and golden brown.

Place tabouhli onto plates and arrange salmon and vegetables over top.

Serves 2

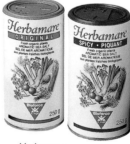

Herbamare

6 baby carrots

2 Belgian endives, cut in half

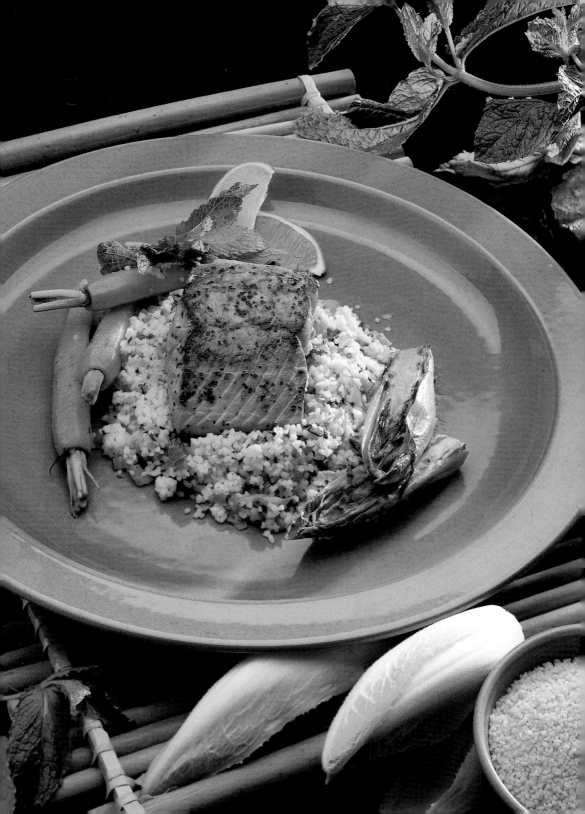

Savoy Cabbage Rolls

Savoy cabbage is the sweetest and tenderest of all cabbages and stuffed with fennel tofu and parsley, makes an unforgettable combination as well as supplies an abundance of phytoestrogens to reduce menopausal discomforts.

6 large leaves Savoy cabbage

2 tbsp cold-pressed olive oil

1 cup (250 ml) **onion, chopped**

2 cloves garlic, minced

1 cup (250 ml) **leek, chopped**

1 cup (250 ml) **organic fermented tofu, finely diced**

1 cup (250 ml) **fennel, finely diced**

1 cup (250 ml) **jicama or pumpkin, finely diced**

1 tsp ginger, minced

1 tbsp parsley, chopped

Sauce:

3 large ripe tomatoes, cut in 1" (2.5 cm) **chunks**

1 tbsp organic butter

2 tbsp onion, chopped

1 clove garlic, minced

Saffron Oil:

Pinch saffron

1 tbsp boiling water

½ cup (125 ml) **extra-virgin olive oil**

To make the sauce, heat butter in a pot over low heat and sauté 2 tablespoons onion and 1 clove minced garlic until tender. Add tomatoes and simmer for 15 minutes or until soft. Place tomato mixture in a blender and blend until smooth. Run through sieve to remove seeds and skin. Return to pot and keep warm.

To make the saffron oil, soak saffron in boiling water for 3 to 4 minutes, then add it to olive oil and let sit for 3 to 4 minutes longer. Strain the saffron.

In the meantime, bring a pot of salted water to a boil and blanch the cabbage leaves for 3 to 4 minutes. Drain and plunge cabbage into ice cold water.

In a saucepan, heat oil and sauté onion, garlic and leek. Add tofu and remaining vegetables and sauté over low heat until soft. Stir in ginger and cilantro.

To assemble the cabbage bundles, lay cabbage leaves on a clean flat surface, fill them with the vegetable mixture and roll. Steam cabbage rolls in a bamboo or vegetable steamer for 5 minutes.

Place cabbage rolls onto plates, drizzle with tomato sauce and saffron oil and serve.

Serves 2

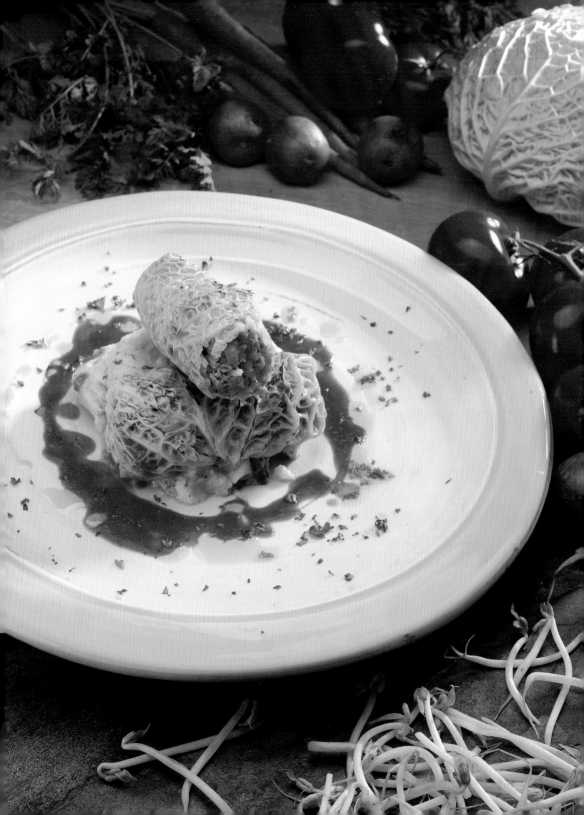

Gratin Pineapple

You can have your dessert and your fiber at the same time! Pineapple is high in fiber and carbohydrates and contains vitamins B complex and C–two important vitamins for supporting the adrenal glands.

1 large fresh pineapple
(about 2 lbs or 900 g)

1 tbsp freshly squeezed lemon juice

1 tbsp sliced almonds, crumbled

1 tsp natural sugar crystals
(see page 42)

1 ½ tbsp cold-pressed pistachio oil

Preheat the oven to 350°F (180°C).

Cut the pineapple into quarters and remove the top ¼" (5 mm) from the core of each piece. Cut the fruit flesh across its width into 1" (2.5 cm) slices, then cut the bottom so that the flesh is separated from the skin, leaving the flesh in the skin. Drizzle with lemon juice and sprinkle with almond and sugar.

Thoroughly wet the pineapple leaves with water and cover them with foil. Set the pineapple in an ovenproof dish and place in the oven for 5 to 7 minutes. Remove from the oven, drizzle pistachio oil over top, and serve.

Serves 4

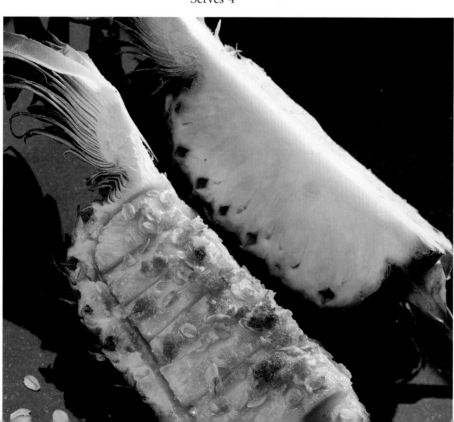

references

Albertazzi, P., et al. "The effect of dietary soy supplementation on hot flushes." Obstetrics and Gynecology 91 (1998): 6-11.

Bruckheim, Allan. The Family Doctor. Portland: Creative Multimedia Corporation, 1992. A textbook on CD-ROM.

Colditz, G.A. "Prospective study of estrogen replacement therapy and risk of breast cancer in postmenopausal women." Journal of the American Medical Association 264 (1990): 2648-2653.

Ewertz, M. "Oral contraceptives and breast cancer risk in Denmark." European Journal of Cancer 28A (6/7) 1992: 1176-1181.

Gaby, Alan R. "Dehydroepiandrosterone: Biological effects and clinical significance." Alternative Medicine Review 1 (2) 1996: 60-69.

Ginsburg, E.S., et al. "Effects of alcohol ingestion on estrogens in postmenopausal women." Journal of the American Medical Association 276 (1996): 1747-1751.

Henrich, J.B. The postmenopausal estrogen/breast cancer controversy. Journal of the American Medical Association 268 (14) 1992:1900-1902.

Lee, John. "Osteoporosis reversal, the role of progesterone." Intern. Clin. Nutr. Rev (1990): 384-391.

Lee, John. "Osteoporosis reversal with transdermal progesterone." Lancet 336 (1990): 1327.

Lee, John. What Your Doctor May Not Tell You About Menopause. New York: Warner Books, 1996.

Rona, Zoltan P., and Jeanne Marie Martin. Return to the Joy of Health. Vancouver: Alive Books, 1995.

Vandenbrouke, J.P. "Postmenopausal estrogen and cardioprotection." Lancet 337 (1991): 833-834.

Wright, Jonathan V., and John Morgenthaler. Natural Hormone Replacement. Petaluma, CA: Smart Publications, 1997.

First published in 2000 by
alive **books**
7436 Fraser Park Drive
Burnaby BC V5J 5B9
(604) 435–1919
1-800–661–0303

© 2000 by *alive* books

Book Design:
  Liza Novecoski
Artwork:
  Terence Yeung
  Raymond Cheung
Food Styling/Recipe Development:
  Fred Edrissi
Photography:
  Edmond Fong (recipe photos)
  Siegfried Gursche
Photo Editing:
  Sabine Edrissi-Bredenbrock
Editing:
  Sandra Tonn
  Marian MacLean

Canadian Cataloguing in Publication Data

Rona MD MSc, Zoltan
  Menopause
  Normally and Naturally

(*alive* natural health guides, 23
ISSN 1490-6503)
ISBN 1-55312-023-X

Printed in Canada

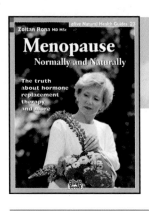

 alive BOOKS

Natural
Your best source of

We hope you enjoyed **Menopause**.
There are 32 other titles to choose from in *alive*'s library
of Natural Health Guides, and more coming soon. The first
series of its kind in North America - now sold on 5 continents!

Self-Help Information

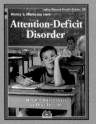 Attention-Deficit Disorder

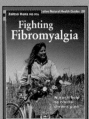 Fighting Fibromyalgia

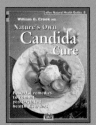 Nature's Own Candida Cure

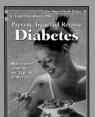 Prevent, Treat and Reverse Diabetes

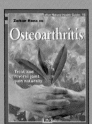 Osteoarthritis

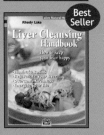 Liver Cleansing Handbook — **Best Seller**

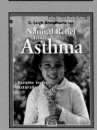 Natural Relief from Asthma

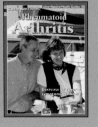 Rheumatoid Arthritis

Healing Foods & Herbs

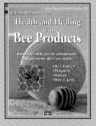 Health and Healing with Bee Products

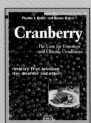 Cranberry

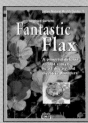 Fantastic Flax

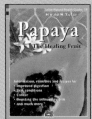 Papaya The Healing Fruit

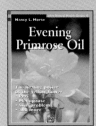 Evening Primrose Oil

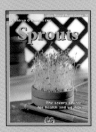 Sprouts

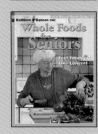 Whole Foods for Seniors

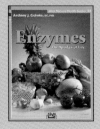 Enzymes

expert authors • easy-to-read information • tasty recipes